Food for Pregnancy Volume 2:

The Moms Guide to Understanding the Best Supplements and Nutrients for a Healthy Growing Baby

MIA ANGELS

Please note the information contained within this document is for educational and entertainment purposes only. Every attempt has been made to provide accurate, up to date and reliable complete information. No warranties of any kind are expressed or implied. Readers acknowledge that the author is not engaging in the rendering of legal, financial, medical or professional advice. The content of this book has been derived from various sources. Please consult a licensed professional before attempting any techniques outlined in this book.

By reading this document, the reader agrees that under no circumstances is the author responsible for any losses, direct or indirect, which are incurred as a result of the use of information contained within this document, including, but not limited to, —errors, omissions, or inaccuracies.

Table of Contents

Introduction

Chapter One: Supplements To Take During Pregnancy

  Why Take Supplements During Pregnancy?

    Pregnancy Increases the Need for Nutrients

    Herbal Supplements During Pregnancy

  Supplements Considered Safe during Pregnancy

    Prenatal Vitamins

    Folate

    Iron

    Vitamin D

    Magnesium

    Ginger

    Fish Oil

    Probiotics

  Supplements to Avoid During Pregnancy

    Vitamin A

    Vitamin E

    Black Cohosh

    Goldenseal

    Dong quai

    Yohimbe

Herbal Supplements Considered Unsafe During Pregnancy

Chapter Two: Anemia in Pregnancy

What Are Red Blood Cells?

What Is Anemia?

Why Do Women Become Anemic During Pregnancy?

Tests for Anemia

Risks Associated With Anemia during Pregnancy

How Can I Avoid Anemia During Pregnancy?

Starting Pregnancy In Great Health

Eating Well During Pregnancy

Supplements

Chapter Three: Bleeding During Pregnancy

Causes Of Bleeding

Changes In The Cervix

'Show'

Placental Abruption

Placenta Praevia

Vasa Praevia

How to Identify the Causes of Bleeding?

Chapter Four: Itching During Pregnancy

Mild itching

Obstetric Cholestasis (OC)

Causes Of Obstetric Cholestasis

Symptoms Of Obstetric Cholestasis

Treating Obstetric Cholestasis

Chapter Five: High Blood Pressure during Pregnancy

Causes of High Blood Pressure during Pregnancy

Risk Factors

Pregnancy

Lifestyle

Age

Different Blood Related Conditions

Chronic hypertension

Gestational hypertension

Superimposed Preeclampsia And Chronic Hypertension

Checking Your Blood Pressure

Normal Blood Pressure

High Blood Pressure

Low Blood Pressure

What Causes Changes in Blood Pressure?

Chapter Six: Preeclampsia

Pre-eclampsia symptoms

Early Symptoms

Progressive Symptoms

How Does Preeclampsia Affect Your Unborn Baby?

Risk factors

Treating preeclampsia

Chapter Seven: Severe Vomiting During Pregnancy

Symptoms of hyperemesis gravidarum

Treating hyperemesis gravidarum

Blood clots and hyperemesis gravidarum

Chapter Eight: Gestational Diabetes During Pregnancy

Symptoms of Gestational Diabetes

What Causes Gestational Diabetes?

Risk Factors for Gestational Diabetes

Gestational Diabetes Tests and Diagnosis

Gestational Diabetes Treatment

Complications of Gestational Diabetes

For The Baby

For the mother

Diet & Exercise

Chapter Nine: Some Other Complications

The Activity Level of the Baby Declines

Early Contractions during the Third Trimester

Water Breaks

Flu Symptoms

Chapter Ten: Exercise and Pregnancy

Exercise tips

Exercises to avoid

Exercises for a fitter pregnancy

Stomach-Strengthening Exercises

Pelvic Tilt Exercises

Pelvic Floor Exercises

Chapter Eleven: Tests from the Lab

Genetic Screening

First Trimester Prenatal Tests

Second Trimester Prenatal Screening Tests

Ultrasound

When Is An Ultrasound Performed During Pregnancy?

First Trimester

Mid-trimester

Third Trimester

Conclusion

Sources

Introduction

Pregnancy is a time of anticipation and excitement, but a few women experience some complications like anemia, high blood pressure or bleeding during their pregnancy. There are several other complications that they may experience during pregnancy.

In the first volume, you learnt about the different nutrients that you must consume during pregnancy, and when you are deficient in any of those nutrients, there are higher chances of there being complications during delivery. Over the course of this book, you will gather information on the different complications that women experience during pregnancy due to deficiencies or otherwise. You will also gather information on what women can do to prevent these complications.

Since most complications arise due to a deficiency in an important nutrient, you will need to take supplements. This book also sheds some light on the different supplements you can take to prevent the deficiency. You will also gather information about the different exercises you can perform to make it easier for you during pregnancy and during birth. It is important that you are cautious when you perform these exercises so you can avoid any complications in the future. There are some tests that you are required to take during your pregnancy to ensure the health of your baby and yourself. These tests have been listed in this book.

Thank you for purchasing the book. I hope you gather all the information you are looking for.

Chapter One: Supplements To Take During Pregnancy

Pregnancy is a very happy experience and one of the most exciting times in a woman's life. However, it can be overwhelming and confusing for some women. Numerous advertisements, magazines and articles on the Internet advise a woman on how she should stay healthy during her pregnancy. Women are aware that they should never smoke, drink alcohol or consume high-mercury seafood during their pregnancy. But few are aware that some vitamins, herbal supplements and minerals must be avoided as well. It becomes very complicated to identify those supplements which are safe and which are not safe to take during pregnancy since this information varies between the sources. This chapter will shed some light on the different supplements that you can take and those you should avoid during your pregnancy.

Why Take Supplements During Pregnancy?

It is important that you consume the right nutrients at every stage of your life, but it is especially important to consume these nutrients during your pregnancy since a pregnant woman will need to nourish their body and also aid in the development of the fetus.

Pregnancy Increases the Need for Nutrients

A woman will need to increase her intake of macronutrients during pregnancy, and these macronutrients include fats, carbohydrates and proteins. This has been covered in detail in the first volume of the book. The requirement of the micronutrients will increase by a large quantity during pregnancy. Vitamins and minerals help to support the fetal and maternal growth at every stage in the pregnancy. These nutrients are important to support some critical functions like cell signaling and cell growth. Some women find it easy to meet these growing needs through their diets, while others cannot. These women will need to take supplements for various reasons including:

1. To prevent nutrient deficiencies, some women may have some deficiencies in the essential vitamins and minerals, and it is important to correct these deficiencies. A shortage in the nutrients can lead to numerous complications during pregnancy and birth defects.
2. To prevent severe vomiting and nausea. This condition is called hyperemesis gravidarum, and can lead to nutrient deficiencies and weight loss.
3. To prevent micronutrient deficiencies caused due to following specific diets. Some women consume a vegan or vegetarian diet because they have some food allergies and intolerances. They need to take supplements to prevent these deficiencies.
4. To cater for the increased need of folate and Vitamin C. Some women find it difficult to quit smoking even during pregnancy, and this will increase their need for folate and vitamin C.
5. To ensure the optimal nutrition for both the mother and her babies if the mother is

carrying more than one baby. When a woman is carrying multiple babies, she will need to increase her nutrient intake so she can provide adequate nutrition to the babies.

6. If a woman consumes a poor diet, or finds it difficult to consume the right foods she will need to take some supplements to avoid any deficiencies in vitamins or minerals.

Some experts from the American Congress of Obstetrics and Gynecology advise all pregnant women to take folic acid supplements and prenatal vitamins during their pregnancy. These supplements will help to prevent any birth defects or deficiencies. It is for this reason that mothers often take supplements.

Herbal Supplements During Pregnancy

During pregnancy, women do not necessarily have to take vitamin or mineral supplements. They can also take herbal supplements. A study found that close to 15.4% women in the US used herbal supplements during their pregnancy.

Close to 25% of these women did not consult their doctors when they were taking these supplements. Some herbal supplements can be taken during pregnancy, but there are others that are bad for women during their pregnancy. Some herbs do help with lowering the risk of complications during pregnancy like an upset stomach or nausea. However, some herbal supplements are harmful for both the mother and the fetus. There is very little research that talks about the benefits of using herbal supplements.

Supplements Considered Safe during Pregnancy

Just like any medication that you take, any herbal or micronutrient supplements you take during your pregnancy should be taken under your doctor's supervision. This is to ensure that you take the supplements in the safe amounts. You should always purchase these supplements from the right brands, so that the supplements are of high quality and are safe to take.

Prenatal Vitamins

Every woman is advised to take prenatal vitamins during her pregnancy, and these vitamins have been formulated to meet the increased demand of these nutrients during pregnancy. These vitamins should be taken before you conceive the baby and during your pregnancy. Some studies show that prenatal vitamins help to reduce the risk of premature birth and preeclampsia. The latter is a dangerous complication that is caused due to high blood pressure and protein in the blood. Prenatal vitamins are not sued to replace a healthy diet, but they will help to prevent any deficiencies since they provide the pregnant woman with the required nutrients. Some prenatal vitamins contain minerals and vitamins that a woman would need to consume during her pregnancy. You will not need to take any other supplements unless advised by your doctor. Some prenatal vitamins that are prescribed by your doctor or midwife will be available over the counter.

Folate

Folate is a Vitamin B, which plays an important role in the synthesis of DNA, production of red blood cells and the growth and development of the fetus. Folic acid is found in many supplements and this is the synthetic form of the folate mineral. This acid will be converted in L-methylfolate, which is the active form of folate. Nutritionists and doctors recommend that women increase their intake of folate up to 600 ug per day. This will help to reduce the risk of developing congenital abnormalities and neural tube defects. Adequate quantities of folate are obtained through the diet, but many women do not eat the required quantity of folate-rich foods. This makes it important for them to take supplements.

Iron

Women will require more iron during their pregnancy since the volume of blood will increase by fifty percent during pregnancy. Iron is a mineral that is essential for the healthy development and growth of the placenta and fetus. This mineral is also important to transfer oxygen throughout the body. Most women are deficient in iron during their pregnancy, and anemia during pregnancy is associated with infant anemia, premature birth and maternal depression. It is recommended that women consume at least 27 mg of iron every day, and women can obtain this amount of iron through prenatal vitamins. Having said that, women with anemia or iron deficiency would need to consume higher doses. If you are not deficient in iron, you should not consume more than the required amount of iron to avoid any side effects including abnormally high hemoglobin levels, constipation and vomiting.

Vitamin D

Vitamin D is a fat-soluble vitamin, which is used by the body to maintain bone health, improve the function of the immune system and aid in cell division. Any deficiency in this vitamin can lead to preeclampsia, gestational diabetes, preterm birth and cesarean section during birth. It is recommended that women take at least 600 IU of Vitamin D per day. Having said that, some experts suggest women require more Vitamin D during their pregnancy. You should always speak to your doctor about your intake of Vitamin D during your pregnancy.

Magnesium

Magnesium is an important mineral that women should consume during their pregnancy. This mineral is an enzyme used in most chemical reactions that take place in your body, and also plays a critical role in nerve, immune and muscle function. If you are deficient in this mineral, it can increase the risk of premature labor and hypertension. Some studies suggest taking magnesium supplements will help to reduce the risk of any complications like premature birth and fetal growth restriction.

Ginger

Ginger is a root that is often used as an herbal supplement and a spice. Ginger is often used as a supplement to reduce nausea, which is caused due to chemotherapy, motion sickness or pregnancy. Ginger is both effective and safe to treat vomiting and nausea that are caused due to pregnancy. Women will be nauseous and vomit during the first trimester, and sometimes they may also experience severe nausea throughout the pregnancy. Ginger will help to reduce this complication, but there is still some research that needs to be conducted to identify the safe dosage of this root.

Fish Oil

If you remember from the first volume, we talked about how fish oil contains the two essential fatty acids EPA and DHA. These oils are important for the development of the brain of the fetus. You can take EPA and DHA supplements to boost the development of the fetus's brain and reduce the risk of maternal depression. There is yet some research that needs to be performed to confirm this. Some studies show EPA and DHA help to improve cognitive function in babies. For instance, one study that was conducted used 2399 women, but there was no difference that could be found in the cognitive development between the infants of mothers who used fish oil supplements and the infants of mothers who did not take any fish oil supplements. This study also concluded that there was no strong effect of this supplement on maternal depression. The study, however, did find that fish oil supplements did help to reduce the risk of premature birth and also helped in the development of the fetus's eyes. It is important for the mother to maintain the required DHA levels in her body to ensure that the fetus develops well. Pregnant women are advised to consume at least two or three servings of low-mercury fish like pollock, sardines and salmon every week.

Probiotics

Since it is important for women to maintain their gut health during their pregnancy, they turn towards probiotics. Probiotics are living microorganisms that benefit the health of the digestive system. Many studies show that it is safe for women to take probiotics during their pregnancy, and there are no side effects that have been identified yet, except for the risk of some infection that can be caused due to probiotics. Numerous studies show supplementing your diet with probiotics will reduce the risk of developing postpartum depression, dermatitis, gestational diabetes and infant eczema. Research is still ongoing on the use of probiotics during pregnancy, and the effects of probiotics on fetal and maternal health are to be discovered.

Supplements to Avoid During Pregnancy

It is important that you supplement your body with some micronutrients or herbs, but there are some that you should avoid.

Vitamin A

Vitamin A is important for the development of the fetus's immune system and vision, but too much Vitamin A can lead to toxicity in the body. The body stores excess Vitamin A in the liver, which accumulates in the body and leads to liver damage. It can also cause some birth defects. For instance, excess amounts of Vitamin A in the body is known to cause some congenital birth defects in babies. Pregnant women will get enough Vitamin A from their diet and through prenatal vitamins, and it is for this reason that they are advised to not take any supplements.

Vitamin E

Vitamin E is a fat-soluble vitamin, which plays numerous roles in the body, and it is involved in improving the function of the immune system and gene expression. This vitamin is important for health, but women are advised to never take vitamin E supplements during their pregnancy. Vitamin E supplements do not improve the health for both the mother and the baby, and can lead to abdominal pain or rupture the amniotic sack.

Black Cohosh

Block cohosh is a plant that is used for numerous reasons including controlling menstrual cramps or hot flashes. This herb is a member of the buttercup family, and it is unsafe to take this herb during pregnancy since it can lead to premature birth or miscarriage because it causes uterine contractions. This herb is also known to cause some liver damage.

Goldenseal

Goldenseal is a plant that is used to treat diarrhea and respiratory infections. It is a dietary supplement, but there is very little evidence that can confirm the safety and the effects of the herb on the body. This herb contains a substance termed berberine, which is known to cause more harm to infants, and can lead to the development of a condition called kernicterus. This condition can lead to brain damage or death. It is for this reason that women are advised to avoid this herb during pregnancy.

Dong quai

Dong quai is a popular medicinal root used in Chinese medicine for over a thousand years. It is used to treat numerous issues right from high blood pressure to menstrual cramps, but there is very little evidence which suggests that this herb is safe to use during pregnancy or even otherwise. It is important that you avoid using this herb during your pregnancy since it can increase the risk of miscarriage since it stimulates uterine contractions.

Yohimbe

Yohimbe is a supplement that is obtained from the bark of a tree native to Africa. This supplement is an herbal remedy used to treat numerous conditions like obesity and erectile dysfunction. It is important that you never use this herb during your pregnancy because it is associated with numerous side effects like heart attacks, seizures and blood pressure.

Herbal Supplements Considered Unsafe During Pregnancy

Some supplements that you should avoid are:

- Red clover
- Saw palmetto
- Pennyroyal
- Tansy
- Wormwood
- Yarrow
- Mugwort
- Blue Cohosh
- Angelica
- Ephedra

Chapter Two: Anemia in Pregnancy

A few women become anemic during their pregnancy. This means that the number of red blood cells decreases in their body. Anemia will make you very tired during your pregnancy, but there are some ways in which you can manage it. If you are anemic during your pregnancy, you will be very tired than usual.

What Are Red Blood Cells?

The cells in your body are called red blood cells, and their role is to transport oxygen through your body. The oxygen is often carried from the heart to your brain, skin, muscles, kidney and every other part of your body. These cells are produced in the marrow in your bones. The red blood cells can carry the oxygen across the body because of the protein hemoglobin. If you want to ensure that you have enough hemoglobin in your body, you will need to consume Vitamin

B12, folate and iron. These nutrients help the body produce the hemoglobin that it needs.

What Is Anemia?

You are anemic if your body does not have the required number of red blood cells in it to carry oxygen to your baby and all around your body. It is common to be mildly anemic during pregnancy, and if you are slightly anemic during pregnancy, you will be a little tired. If you have severe anemia, you will constantly be out of breath and will be terribly weak, irritable, and dizzy and may also find it very hard to concentrate on any task that you are performing. You will also find that your heart races every time.

Why Do Women Become Anemic During Pregnancy?

When a woman is pregnant, her body will change. These changes are necessary for promoting the growth of the baby. When you are pregnant, your body will need to make a lot more blood. A woman who is not pregnant will have close to five liters of blood in her body, but when she is pregnant, she will have at least eight liters of blood in her body. The body needs a lot of folate, iron and Vitamin B12 to increase the number of cells in the body, and also produce the extra hemoglobin. Anemia is mainly caused due to iron deficiency during pregnancy. When you are pregnant, you must remember to consume at least three times the amount of iron that you would consume when you are menstruating. It is unfortunately hard for the body to absorb iron, and this makes it harder to produce hemoglobin. It is for this reason that women are at a higher risk of being anemic during pregnancy.

Tests for Anemia

When you find out you are pregnant and go to visit the doctor or midwife, you will be asked to take a blood test which will help them understand your hemoglobin level. If there are any abnormalities in this test, you may need to take more tests to check the levels of folate, iron and Vitamin B12 in your body. You may also need to take a few tests that will shed some light on inherited disorders.

Risks Associated With Anemia during Pregnancy

Most women are tired during their pregnancy, but anemia worsens this condition. It will make you feel breathless and tired. The probability of you requiring a blood transfusion once you give birth to your baby will increase. Anemia can increase the risk of low birth weight and premature birth, and there is also a possibility that your child may be anemic.

How Can I Avoid Anemia During Pregnancy?

You can avoid anemia during pregnancy in the following ways:

- Always start your pregnancy in good health
- Make sure that you eat the right foods during pregnancy
- Take supplements if required

Starting Pregnancy In Great Health

If you are trying to become pregnant, you should first meet with your doctor and get a full body check-up done. You will need to ask your doctor to shed some light on some conditions like anemia, and also ask your doctor about the supplements you may need to take for folate. Doctors often advise women to take a folate supplement for one month before they become pregnant, and continue to take that supplement until the end of the first trimester. This helps to reduce the risk of spina bifida and other neural tube defects. Women are advised to take at least 0.5 milligrams of folic acid every day during their pregnancy, but this amount varies if the woman is pregnant. Ensure that you always discuss your conditions with your doctor to avoid worsening the situation.

Eating Well During Pregnancy

As mentioned in the first volume of the book, it is important that you eat the right food. You can lower the risk of being anemic by consuming foods that are rich in iron, like iron fortified cereals and breads, spinach, egg, dried fruit and meat. Vitamin B12 is found in dairy products, eggs, shellfish, meat and fish. Leafy green vegetables, muesli, beans, beef, broccoli, asparagus and Brussels sprouts are rich in folic acid, and it is advised that you consume these foods to lower the risk of anemia. If you are a vegetarian, you should replace the meat and fish with beans, lentils, soymilk, eggs and tofu. You should also meet with a dietician to learn more about how you can improve your nutrition, and also gather information about the different supplements you may need to take. It is best to avoid tea and coffee immediately after a meal, and also consume citrus fruit to improve your body's ability to absorb the iron that is found in the food you consume. This will help to prevent anemia.

Supplements

Women are advised to take some supplements for folic acid during their pregnancy, and they are also advised to consume food that is rich in folate. Many women are required to take iron supplements especially when they are at a higher risk of becoming deficient or are deficient. Vegans and vegetarians are often asked to take supplements for the B12 vitamin, and if you have been asked to take those supplements you should speak to your doctor to learn about the side effects of supplements, and what you should do to avoid them.

Chapter Three: Bleeding During Pregnancy

It is common for women to bleed during their pregnancy, but any signs of vaginal bleeding are dangerous. If you notice that you are bleeding from the vagina, you should consult your doctor or midwife immediately. It is important to identify the cause of bleeding immediately, although it is not caused because of any serious issues. If you notice that you are bleeding from your vagina, you should contact your doctor immediately. There is a possibility that you may have some light bleeding during the first few weeks into your pregnancy, and this is called spotting. You bleed at this time since the fetus would have planted itself in the walls of the uterus. This bleeding is also termed as implantation bleeding, and will happen around the time of the first period after you have conceived.

Causes Of Bleeding

Vaginal bleeding during the first two months of pregnancy can be a sign of ectopic pregnancy or miscarriage. Ectopic pregnancy is the condition where the fetus implants itself in the fallopian tube. That said, many women who have had vaginal bleeding during this stage do have successful pregnancies and give birth to healthy babies. Vaginal bleeding can be caused due to other causes during the next few months of pregnancy. Some of the causes have been listed in this section.

Changes In The Cervix

If you have sex during pregnancy, the cells in the cervix will change. They will become more sensitive and can cause bleeding. This condition is called cervical ectropion, which is a harmless condition. Quite often you may develop vaginal infections, which can lead to bleeding.

'Show'

Show is the small quantity of blood that is mixed with the mucus. Most women have this sort of bleeding in the last trimester. During pregnancy, there is a plug of mucus that covers or seals the cervix. The mucus will mix with the blood when the plug comes away. This means that the cells in the cervix are changing, and your body is getting ready to enter the first stages of labor. This type of bleeding will occur either during labor or a few days before you go into labor.

Placental Abruption

Placental Abruption is a very serious condition where the placenta will start to come away from the wall of the womb. This condition does not necessarily lead to vaginal bleeding, but will cause a stomach pain. You may give birth to your baby earlier if this condition occurs a few days before the due date.

Placenta Praevia

Placenta Praevia, also termed low-lying placenta is a condition where the placenta is very close to the cervix or covering it, since it is attached to the lower section of the womb. This will make it difficult for your baby to come out of your body. You can check the position of your placenta in the morphology scan. The baby will not be able to move past the placenta if it is covering or close to the cervix. In these conditions, the doctor will recommend that you have a caesarean.

Vasa Praevia

Vasa Praevia is a condition that occurs when the blood vessels in the umbilical cord cover the service through the membranes. This condition occurs in about 1 in 3000 to 1 in 6000 births. The blood vessels in the umbilical cord are often protected within the membrane of the cord, but if the membrane ruptures and your water breaks at the same time, these vessels can tear. This will lead to vaginal bleeding, and there is a chance that your baby may lose a lot of blood and die. It is difficult to identify the symptoms of vasa Praevia that makes it hard to diagnose. That being said, an ultrasound could help to spot this condition before birth. If the baby's heart rate suddenly changes, either drops or becomes rapid, or there is some bleeding in the vagina, you should ask your doctor to check for vasa

Praevia. This condition is linked with placenta Praevia.

How to Identify the Causes of Bleeding?

You will need to have an ultrasound scan, a vaginal or pelvic examination or a blood test to check the hormone levels to identify the reason behind vaginal bleeding. You will also be asked about some other symptoms like dizziness, pain, cramps and more. If your baby is not due for a long time and the symptoms are not severe, the doctor will monitor you and may keep you under observation for a few days. Depending on what is causing the bleeding, you may need to stay in the hospital only for one night or until you give birth. This is to keep you and your baby healthy, and deliver your baby safely regardless of what the situation may be.

Chapter Four: Itching During Pregnancy

You may have some mild itching during your pregnancy since your blood will supply more blood to the skin. The skin around your abdomen will also be stretched during your pregnancy as your baby grows, and this may also feel slightly itchy. You do not have to worry about mild itching, but if the itching becomes severe it could be a sign of obstetric cholestasis, which is a liver condition. Only one pregnant woman out of 100 will be affected by this condition.

Mild itching

You can wear loose clothes to prevent any itching since your clothes will not cause any friction by rubbing against your skin. This will reduce any irritation. You should try to wear only cotton or other natural fabrics to ensure that air will circulate across your body. You may also feel relief when you apply some moisturizer or lotion or take a cool bath. If you find that some strong perfumes irritate your skin, you should switch to mild perfumes. If you have severe itching, which does not stop, you should consult your doctor immediately.

Obstetric Cholestasis (OC)

Obstetric cholestasis (OC) or intrahepatic cholestasis is a liver disorder, which only affects some women during pregnancy, especially in the last trimester.

Causes Of Obstetric Cholestasis

The causes of OC are still unclear. In some cases, the pregnancy hormone can also be involved. Since the pregnancy hormones increase in the body during pregnancy, these hormones will reduce the flow of bile. This means that the number of salts in the bile will add up in the liver instead of leaving it. These salts will enter the bloodstream, which will make you feel itchy.

OC often runs in families, but it can occur during pregnancy even if you do not have any family that has been affected by this disorder. If you did have OC in a previous pregnancy, you may also develop it during your subsequent pregnancies. If you have OC, the risk of premature birth and stillbirth increases. Your baby may also have some issues with breathing, and your doctor may induce labor even before your due date to prevent these complications.

Symptoms Of Obstetric Cholestasis

One of the classic symptoms of OC is an itch without any rash. This usually happens on the soles of your feet and your palms, but some times it can be more widespread. The itching will become worse at night and is also unbearable and continuous. Another symptom of OC is jaundice, pale bowel movements and dark urine. You will find that the itchiness has gone after you gave birth.

Treating Obstetric Cholestasis

Obstetric cholestasis can be diagnosed based on family and medical history. You can also take some blood tests to check the functioning of the liver. If you are diagnosed with OG, you will need to have liver function tests regularly until you give birth. These tests will allow the doctor to closely monitor your condition. Calamine lotion and other creams prescribed by your doctor can be used during pregnancy. These creams can provide some relief. Your doctor may also ask you to take some medication that reduces itching and decreases the number of bile salts. OC will make it difficult for your body to absorb Vitamin K, which is an important nutrient to ensure that blood clots. Discuss your options and your health with your doctor or midwife if you are diagnosed with OC.

Chapter Five: High Blood Pressure during Pregnancy

It is said that you have high blood pressure if the measure of your blood pressure is either equal to or greater than 130/80 mm Hg. This condition is serious and is a major concern for many women. If it is managed well, high blood pressure does not necessarily have to be dangerous during pregnancy.

Causes of High Blood Pressure during Pregnancy

There are numerous reasons why a woman may develop high blood pressure during her pregnancy, and these include:

- Being obese or overweight
- Not keeping yourself active
- Drinking alcohol

- Smoking
- First-time pregnancy
- History of hypertension in the family
- Age is over 35
- Multiple births
- Having autoimmune diseases like diabetes

Risk Factors

There are some risk factors that lead to high blood pressure during pregnancy.

Pregnancy

Women who are pregnant for the first time will most likely have high blood pressure, but there is a chance that this condition will not arise during future pregnancies. If a woman is carrying multiple babies, it can lead to hypertension. The woman's body will need to twice or thrice as hard to ensure that it provides the required nourishment to the babies.

Lifestyle

An unhealthy lifestyle can increase the risk of developing hypertension or high blood pressure during pregnancy. If you are obese or overweight, or not keeping yourself active, the risk of developing high blood pressure will increase.

Age

Pregnant women who are above the age of thirty-five are at a higher risk of developing hypertension. Women who have hypertension before they become pregnant will be at a higher risk of developing some complications during pregnancy when compared to those women who have normal blood pressure before they become pregnant.

Different Blood Related Conditions

There are three different conditions that a woman can develop during pregnancy if she has hypertension.

Chronic hypertension

Many times women have hypertension or high blood pressure before they become pregnant. This condition is also known as chronic hypertension and can be treated with medication. Doctors also say that women who develop hypertension during their pregnancy have chronic hypertension, and this is true for those women who develop hypertension during the first twenty weeks of their pregnancy.

Gestational hypertension

You can develop gestational hypertension during your twentieth week of pregnancy, and this condition will resolve after delivery. If gestational hypertension is diagnosed before thirty weeks, it can increase the risk of developing preeclampsia.

Superimposed Preeclampsia And Chronic Hypertension

If you had chronic hypertension before you became pregnant, you will develop preeclampsia during your pregnancy. This can lead to some additional complications during pregnancy including protein in your urine.

Checking Your Blood Pressure

The blood pressure is measured as a fraction where the systolic blood pressure is the numerator and the diastolic blood pressure is the denominator. The systolic blood pressure will measure the pressure of blood in your arteries when your heart is squeezing or beating the blood from the heart to your body. The diastolic pressure will measure the pressure of blood in your arteries when your heart is at rest.

You do not have to go to the doctor to track your blood pressure, but can purchase a blood pressure monitor online or from the pharmacy. Most of these devices will be placed only on your upper arm or wrist. You can take the monitor to your doctor's office to help you check the accuracy of the monitor. You can also visit any store including a grocery store or pharmacy where you can take the blood pressure readings. You should take the readings of the blood pressure at the same time every day to ensure that you have accurate readings. Keep your legs uncrossed and always use the same arm. If you have high blood pressure repeatedly, you should inform your doctor immediately.

Normal Blood Pressure

Your doctor will take a baseline measurement of your blood pressure at the start of your pregnancy to determine what your normal blood pressure during pregnancy should be. They will then measure the blood pressure during every visit.

High Blood Pressure

If your blood pressure is greater than 130/99 mm Hg, or you are at a higher number than the pressure before you became pregnant, you will need to visit the doctor immediately. High blood pressure is defined as a high systolic with a diastolic that is 90 mm Hg or higher or the pressure is 140 mm Hg. The blood pressure may decrease for a woman early in pregnancy, since the pregnancy hormones will lead to the widening of the blood vessels, and as a result of this the flow of blood in the body will not be too high.

Low Blood Pressure

There is no number that you can put to determine low blood pressure. The following are some symptoms of low blood pressure:

- Cold and clammy skin
- Headache
- Feeling Faint
- Dizziness
- Nausea

What Causes Changes in Blood Pressure?

When a woman progresses through her pregnancy, the blood pressure can return to the normal level or change depending on your body. Here are some reasons behind why this may happen.

1. The quantity of blood will increase in the body. Numerous studies conclude that a woman's blood volume will increase by forty-five percent during pregnancy, and this extra blood will need to be pumped throughout the body by the heart.
2. The left side of the heart, which does the pumping, will become larger and thicker. This will give the heart a chance to pump more blood.
3. The kidneys will increase the production of the hormone vasopressin, which will lead to water retention in the body.

High blood pressure during pregnancy will often reduce when you give birth to the baby. In some situations, the blood pressure will continue to be elevated and your doctor will prescribe some medication to bring the level back to normal.

Chapter Six: Preeclampsia

Many women develop preeclampsia during their pregnancy after twenty weeks. They may also develop preeclampsia immediately after they deliver their baby. If you have preeclampsia, you will have fluid retention or edema, high blood pressure and some protein in the urine. If you do not treat this immediately, it can lead to some severe complications, and can be life threatening in some instances. Preeclampsia can lead to growth and development problems in the baby.

The exact cause of preeclampsia is still unknown, but it is thought that preeclampsia occurs whenever there is an issue with the placenta. Women may not realize that they have preeclampsia during their pregnancy, and it can only be diagnosed through routine appointments with the doctor or midwife.

Pre-eclampsia symptoms

Early Symptoms

Women who develop preeclampsia will show the following symptoms:

- Protein in the urine or proteinuria
- Hypertension or high blood pressure

You will not notice these symptoms during your pregnancy, but your midwife or doctor should pick these up during your appointments. Most pregnant women suffer from high blood pressure, so this cannot suggest preeclampsia. If there is protein in your urine, it can be used to indicate the condition.

Progressive Symptoms

When you develop preeclampsia, it will lead to retention of fluid. This will cause swelling in the ankles, feet, hands and face. Fluid retention or edema is a common symptom of pregnancy, but it will only happen in the lower parts of the body like the ankles and the feet. Edema will gradually develop, but if the swelling is very sudden it can be a sign of preeclampsia. Preeclampsia may cause the following as it progresses:

- Less urine
- Vision problems, such as seeing flashing lights or blurring
- Feeling generally unwell
- Nausea and vomiting
- Excessive weight gain
- Dizziness
- Severe headaches
- Shortness of breath
- Pain in the upper abdomen (just below the ribs)

When you notice any of these symptoms, you should meet your doctor immediately. Preeclampsia can lead to numerous complications if it is not treated properly. Some of these complications are:

- HELLP (a combination of blood-clotting and liver disorder)
- Stroke

- Eclampsia (convulsions)
- Problems in the kidneys and brain

These complications are, however, extremely rare.

How Does Preeclampsia Affect Your Unborn Baby?

Preeclampsia can lead to premature birth of your baby, and one of the main signs of preeclampsia is slow growth of the fetus. The fetus will not receive adequate blood supply through the placenta, and the fetus will also receive fewer nutrients and less oxygen, which are essential for the growth of the baby. This condition is termed as intra-uterine growth retardation or intra-uterine growth restriction.

Risk factors

Some factors have been identified which can increase the risk of developing preeclampsia. Some of them are:

- You developed preeclampsia during your previous pregnancy which means that there is a twenty percent probability that you will develop this condition in future pregnancies.
- You have high blood pressure, migraines, diabetes and kidney disease.

Some of the other risk factors are:

- There are higher chances of you developing preeclampsia during your first pregnancy when compared to your future pregnancies.
- Your last pregnancy was over ten years ago.
- Either your mother or sister had preeclampsia during their pregnancy.
- You are either aged over 40 or are a teenager.
- You were obese before your pregnancy.
- You are having twins or triplets.

Treating preeclampsia

You can treat preeclampsia by maintaining your blood pressure and treating the other symptoms through medication. One of the simplest ways to treat preeclampsia is to give birth to the baby.

Chapter Seven: Severe Vomiting During Pregnancy

Vomiting and nausea are very common during pregnancy, and this is especially true during the first trimester. Some women experience excessive vomiting and nausea, and this condition is called hyperemesis gravidarum. You will need to be treated by a doctor if you suffer from this condition. This condition is not very common, but it can be treated. It is worse than morning sickness, and if you are unable to keep any food or fluids down, you should tell your doctor or midwife immediately.

Symptoms of hyperemesis gravidarum

If you have excessive vomiting during your pregnancy, you will find that it is much worse than morning sickness or nausea. The symptoms of excessive vomiting will start five weeks into your pregnancy, and will resolve by the twentieth week. Some of the signs of hyperemesis gravidarum are:

- Ketosis, which is a serious condition that is caused due to an increase in the number of ketones in the urine and blood. Ketones are acidic chemicals that are produced by your body when it breaks down fat to produce energy.
- Severe or prolonged vomiting and nausea
- Weight loss
- Dehydration
- Confusion, jaundice, fainting and headaches
- Hypotension or low blood pressure when you stand up

The vomiting or nausea is often so severe that it becomes impossible for you to keep any food or fluids in your stomach. This will lead to weight loss and dehydration. Hyperemesis gravidarum is often unpleasant and has some dramatic symptoms. The good news is that it will not harm your baby. That being said, if you lose too much weight during pregnancy there is a risk of low birth weight.

Treating hyperemesis gravidarum

Some cases of hyperemesis gravidarum can be controlled using antacids, through rest and through a change in diet. Some severe cases of hyperemesis gravidarum will require special treatment, and you will need to be admitted in the hospital so that your doctor can asses the condition and give you the required treatment. You may be given some intravenous fluids through a drip to stop the vomiting and also treat the ketosis. You should never take any medication without speaking to your doctor first.

Blood clots and hyperemesis gravidarum

Since hyperemesis gravidarum can lead to dehydration, you are at a higher risk of developing a blood clot or deep being thrombosis.

Chapter Eight: Gestational Diabetes During Pregnancy

If you have high levels of blood sugar during your pregnancy, you have gestational diabetes. Your blood sugar levels may have been normal before you became pregnant, but they may have increased during your pregnancy. Having said that, you could still give birth to a healthy baby even if you have gestational diabetes. You should visit your doctor and take some simple steps that will help you manage your blood sugar levels. When you baby is born, you will see that the gestational diabetes goes away. The risk of developing Type II diabetes after you give birth increases if you have gestational diabetes.

Symptoms of Gestational Diabetes

There are no symptoms of gestational diabetes in women, and many women only learn that they have gestational diabetes when they go through their routine tests.

What Causes Gestational Diabetes?

The placenta produces hormones during pregnancy, and these hormones can increase the quantity of glucose in your blood. The pancreas will produce enough insulin, which can handle this increase in glucose, but if your body cannot produce the required quantity of insulin, the blood sugar levels will increase. This will lead to the development of gestational diabetes.

Risk Factors for Gestational Diabetes

Gestational diabetes affects at least ten percent of pregnancy each year, and you may develop gestational diabetes if you:

- Are Asian, African-American, Native American or Hispanic
- Were overweight before you were pregnant
- Have a family history of diabetes
- Have very high blood sugar levels, but this does not necessarily lead to diabetes
- Have some medical complications including high blood pressure
- Have given birth to a baby who weighed greater than nine pounds
- Have given birth to a baby with birth defects or a stillborn baby
- Are older than 25
- Have had gestational diabetes in previous pregnancies

Gestational Diabetes Tests and Diagnosis

It is only after twelve weeks that the risk of gestational diabetes will increase. Your doctor will check your blood sugar levels to identify if you have gestational diabetes after the twenty-fourth week of pregnancy. If you are at a higher risk, you will need to get tested sooner. Before you go for a gestational diabetes test, you should first drink a drink that is filled with sugar. This will increase the levels of blood sugar in your body. You should take a blood test an hour later to understand how your body has handled the large quantities of sugar. If your test results show that your blood sugar levels are higher than the required cutoff, you will need to conduct more tests. This will mean that you should test the blood sugar when you fast and also take a glucose test after three hours. You may need to take another test later during your pregnancy even if your test results are normal, but you are at a higher risk of developing gestational diabetes.

Gestational Diabetes Treatment

Your doctor will ask you to do the following when you want to treat gestational diabetes:

- Get urine tests done to check the level of ketones in your body

- Always check your levels of blood sugar at least four times a day
- Consume a healthy diet
- Always exercise

Your doctor will constantly track your weight gain, and will also let you know if there is any other medicine that you will need to take to treat gestational diabetes.

Complications of Gestational Diabetes

There are many other complications that can arise because of gestational diabetes.

For The Baby

- Type 2 diabetes later in life
- Early birth
- High birth weight
- Low blood sugar
- Respiratory distress syndrome

For the mother

- Diabetes later in life
- Diabetes in a future pregnancy
- High blood pressure and preeclampsia
- Higher chance of C-section

If you want to prevent gestational diabetes or develop diabetes in the future, you should begin getting yourself tested for diabetes at least eight weeks after you give birth.

Diet & Exercise

Follow the steps mentioned below to prevent gestational diabetes:

- Eat a low-sugar and healthy diet. Ask your nutritionist to develop a meal plan that is prepared for someone who has diabetes. You should switch to natural foods like carrots, raisins and fruit instead of consuming candy, ice cream and cookies. You should also increase your intake of whole grains and vegetables, and watch the size of your servings.

- You should never lose weight during your pregnancy, so if you are overweight try to lose weight before you become pregnant. You should ensure that you are at the ideal weight before you become pregnant.
- Ensure that you always exercise during your pregnancy. If you are trying to conceive, you should begin exercising then. Try to exercise for at least thirty minutes every day.
- You should also ensure that you obtain the appropriate prenatal care. You should take all the necessary tests when you are pregnant, and ensure that you speak to your doctor about your food and your activity.

Chapter Nine: Some Other Complications

There are some other complications that you should be aware of during your pregnancy.

The Activity Level of the Baby Declines

If your baby was previously active, but seems to have less energy now you need not worry. This can be normal, but how will you be able to tell? You can try a few things before you rush to the doctor to understand if there is a problem. Either eat something or drink something cold, and lie on your side. If your baby moves now, you do not have to worry. You should also count the number of times your baby kicks you. You should always set a benchmark of your baby's activity to understand whether your baby is moving less or more. Your baby should kick you at least ten times in two hours, and if he or she kicks lesser number of times, you will need to consult your doctor. Alternatively, you can take an ultrasound to determine the growth and development of the fetus.

Early Contractions during the Third Trimester

Early contractions are a sign of premature birth. Many first-time mothers cannot differentiate between false labor and true labor. False labor contractions or Braxton-Hicks contractions are non-rhythmic and unpredictable. They also do not increase in intensity. If you drink enough water, these contractions will subside in a few hours. Regular contractions, however, will increase in intensity and they are about ten minutes apart. If you are in your third trimester and you have contractions, you should call the doctor right away. Your doctor can stop the labor if it is too early for your baby to come out.

Water Breaks

You feel water rushing down your legs when you got up from the couch to grab a glass of water. You may think that your water has broken, but it could be urine leakage too. Your bladder is under a lot of pressure during your pregnancy because of the enlarged uterus. It is only for a few women that water breaking will be a dramatic gush of fluid.

You should go to the bathroom immediately and empty your bladder if you are not sure why there is a sudden gush of fluid. If the fluid does not stop, you could have broken your water, and you should go to the hospital.

Flu Symptoms

Experts say that women should always get the flu vaccine during their pregnancy. Women are more likely to get sick during pregnancy, and have some serious complications that are caused by the flu. If you do get the flu, do not rush to the hospital. Talk to your doctor first and see what you can do.

Chapter Ten: Exercise and Pregnancy

It is important that you perform regular physical activity during your pregnancy since this has multiple benefits. Physical activity will also prepare your body for childbirth. It is important that you understand your body and choose the right exercises to keep you strong. You can modify these exercises to make it easier for you. You do not have to perform strenuous exercises during pregnancy. You must be sensible about the level of exercise that you are performing. You must consult a healthcare professional, doctor, physiotherapist or your midwife to ensure that your exercise routine is not harmful for you or the baby.

Exercise tips

You should never exhaust yourself. Try to perform light exercises during your pregnancy. You will need to reduce the number of exercises you perform and slow down as your pregnancy progresses. If you are ever in doubt, you should consult your doctor or midwife. One way to measure whether the exercise is light or moderate is to see whether you can have a conversation while you exercise. You are probably exercising too much if you are unable to maintain a conversation while you exercise.

If you were never active before you were pregnant, do not take up strenuous exercises immediately. Regardless of the type of exercise you take up, you should let the instructor know that you are pregnant. Make sure that you do not perform more than fifteen minutes of exercise continuously. You can increase the time you spend on exercising to thirty minutes when you feel better. Remember that exercise only should be beneficial and not strenuous.

Some tips that you should keep in mind are:

- Always perform some warm-up and cool-down exercises.
- Try to stay active for at least thirty minutes every day. You can walk for thirty

minutes or perform any small exercise for thirty minutes.

- Do not perform any strenuous exercises during humid or hot weather.
- Always drink plenty of water.
- Ensure that your instructor is qualified and is aware that you are pregnant.
- Swimming is a good exercise to consider since the water will support the weight of your fetus.

Exercises to avoid

- After 16 weeks of gestation, you should avoid lying down on your back since the weight of your bump will press against some blood vessels which will reduce the flow of blood to the fetus and also make you feel weak or faint.
- Avoid any kind of contact sports since there is a risk of you being hit. Do not participate in activities like judo, rugby, football, tennis, squash or kickboxing.
- Avoid downhill skiing, horse riding, cycling, gymnastics and ice hockey since there is a possibility that you may fall.

- Since the fetus does not have any protection from gas embolism or decompression sickness, you should avoid scuba diving.
- You should avoid going to heights above 2,500 meters unless you are acclimatized to the weather conditions in those areas.

Exercises for a fitter pregnancy

You should try to perform the exercises during your pregnancy. These exercises will help to strengthen the muscles in your back and pelvis, allowing you to carry the extra weight. They will also help to improve circulation, make your joints stronger, ease your backache and make you feel better.

Stomach-Strengthening Exercises

When your baby starts growing bigger, you will find that the lower back has a hollow, and this will increase during the pregnancy. This will give you a backache and make it difficult for you to stand. You should perform some abdominal muscle exercises to strength the muscles and ease your backache.

- Lower yourself carefully to the ground and place your hands on your shoulders and knees under the hips.
- Keep your back straight and stretch your fingers forward.
- Take a deep breath in and pull the muscles of your stomach towards your back.
- Now, raise your back up and move your head towards the ceiling. Let your head relax. Ensure that you do not lock your elbows.
- Hold this position for four seconds and move back to the center.
- You must ensure that you do not bend your back. Always keep your back straight. Perform this exercise ten times and make sure that you move the muscles carefully.
- Do not exert yourself or push yourself. Let your back move only as much as it can.

Pelvic Tilt Exercises

- Stand against a wall with your legs shoulder-width apart.
- Slightly bend your knees.
- Breathe in deeply and pull your stomach in towards your spine. Flatten your back against the wall and hold your breath for four seconds. Exhale softly.
- Repeat this exercise ten times.

Pelvic Floor Exercises

Pelvic floor exercises will help to strengthen the muscles on your pelvis. These muscles are under great stress and strain during pregnancy and birth. The pelvis consists of numerous layers of muscles that will stretch to create some support from the end of the backbone to the pubic bone.

Chapter Eleven: Tests from the Lab

You will be asked to take numerous tests, imaging and screenings during your pregnancy, and these tests are designed to help you and the doctor assess the health of your baby. Your doctor will use these tests to optimize the prenatal development and care that you provide to your baby.

Genetic Screening

It is easy to diagnose different types of genetic abnormalities before you give birth to your baby. Your midwife or doctor may ask you to take some genetic tests during your pregnancy if either you or your partner has had a history of different genetic disorders. If you were pregnant with a baby who had a genetic abnormality while still in the womb, it is always a good to take a genetic screening to protect your baby.

Some genetic disorders that can be diagnosed before birth are:

- Hemophilia A
- Sickle cell disease
- Cystic fibrosis
- Thalassemia
- Polycystic kidney disease
- Duchenne muscular dystrophy
- Tay-Sachs disease

You can use the screening methods mentioned below during your pregnancy:

- Amniocentesis
- Alpha-fetoprotein (AFP) test or multiple marker test
- Cell-free fetal DNA testing
- Percutaneous umbilical blood sampling (taking a small sample of the baby's blood from the umbilical cord)
- Chorionic villus sampling
- Ultrasound scan

First Trimester Prenatal Tests

During the first trimester, you will need to take a maternal blood test and an ultrasound to check the fetus's development. These tests will help the doctor determine if the fetus is at a risk of developing any birth defects. The screening tests performed during the first trimester include:

1. Ultrasound to determine nuchal translucency: This test will examine the area around the fetus's neck to check for thickening or increased fluid through an ultrasound.
2. Ultrasound to determine the nasal bone: It is difficult to view the nasal bone in some babies who have a chromosome abnormality like Down syndrome. An ultrasound is performed during the eleventh week of gestation to determine the nasal bone.
3. Maternal blood or serum tests: These tests are used to measure the levels of two substances that are found in every pregnant woman:
    a. Plasma Protein A: This protein is produced in the first few weeks into

pregnancy in the placenta, and abnormal levels of this protein will increase the risk of chromosomal abnormality.

b. Chorionic Gonadotropin: This hormone is also produced in the placenta during the first few weeks into pregnancy, and abnormal levels of this hormone will increase the risk of chromosomal abnormality.

If the results of any of these tests are abnormal, it is important that you seek genetic counseling. Some additional tests like amniocentesis, chorionic villus sampling, ultrasounds and fetal DNA tests will need to be completed to accurately diagnose the issues.

Second Trimester Prenatal Screening Tests

During the second trimester, you will need to take several tests called multiple markers. These tests provide information about any birth defects or genetic disorders that your baby may develop during the pregnancy. These tests are conducted by taking a blood sample between your sixteenth and eighteenth week of pregnancy. Some of these markers include:

1. AFP screening: This test will measure the levels of the serum AFP in your blood during your pregnancy. AFP is a protein that is produced by the amniotic fluid that covers the fetus, and this protein can enter your blood when it passes through the placenta. If your blood has abnormal levels of AFP, it can indicate the following:
   a. Defects in the wall of the abdomen in the fetus
   b. Since the levels are different throughout the pregnancy, it can indicate a miscalculated due date
   c. Chromosomal abnormalities like Down syndrome
   d. Spina bifida and other neural tube defects
   e. Twins – in this instance, the higher levels of AFP in your blood are because two fetuses are producing the same protein

2. Estriol, inhibin and chorionic gonadotropin are hormones that can be used to determine the health of the fetus. This hormone is produced in the placenta.

Any abnormal results in these tests mean that some additional testing will need to be done to eliminate doubt. Your doctor may ask you to take an ultrasound to check the health of the fetus and also reassess the milestones of your pregnancy. When you have performed the tests during your first and second trimester, you can use the results to confirm whether your fetus is healthy or not.

Ultrasound

An ultrasound scan is used to create an image of the baby and the internal organs using high-frequency sound waves. An ultrasound is performed during your pregnancy to verify the due date and check the growth of the fetus.

When Is An Ultrasound Performed During Pregnancy?

An ultrasound is performed during the pregnancy for numerous reasons:

First Trimester

- Detect any abnormalities in the fetus
- Examine the anatomy of the uterus
- Determine the number of fetuses
- Assess the due date
- Diagnose miscarriage or ectopic pregnancy

Mid-trimester

- Reassess the due date if necessary
- Assist in some prenatal tests
- Examine the fetus for abnormalities if any
- Check the quantity of amniotic fluid
- Monitor the growth of the fetus
- Examine the flow of blood
- Observe fetal activity and behavior
- Measure the length of the cervix

Third Trimester

- Monitor the growth of the fetus
- Check the quantity of amniotic fluid
- Assess the placenta
- Determine the position of the fetus
- Conduct a biophysical profile test

Conclusion

Thank you for purchasing the book.

Pregnancy is one of the most exciting times of a woman's life, but it is also one of the most sensitive periods of her life. A woman will need to take numerous things into account with respect to her nutrition to ensure that she and her baby are safe. Over the course of this book, you will gather information on different supplements you can take to prevent deficiencies and different complications during pregnancy. I hope you gather all the information you are looking for and are healthy during your pregnancy.

Sources

https://www.webmd.com/baby/features/7-pregnancy-warning-signs#2

https://www.pregnancybirthbaby.org.au/search-results/complications

https://www.healthline.com/health/pregnancy/delivery-complications#risk-factors

https://www.pregnancybirthbaby.org.au/pregnancy-complications

https://www.pregnancybirthbaby.org.au/severe-vomiting-during-pregnancy-hyperemesis-gravidarum

https://www.pregnancybirthbaby.org.au/bleeding-during-pregnancy

https://www.pregnancybirthbaby.org.au/itching
-during-pregnancy

https://www.pregnancybirthbaby.org.au/pre-
eclampsia

https://www.healthline.com/nutrition/supplem
ents-during-pregnancy#TOC_TITLE_HDR_5

https://www.healthline.com/health/high-blood-
pressure-hypertension/during-
pregnancy#complications

https://www.webmd.com/diabetes/gestational-
diabetes#2

https://www.pregnancybirthbaby.org.au/exercis
ing-during-pregnancy

https://www.hopkinsmedicine.org/health/welln
ess-and-prevention/common-tests-during-
pregnancy